The
Productivity Rocket

Turn Your Personal Effectiveness into a Lifetime Habit

*****

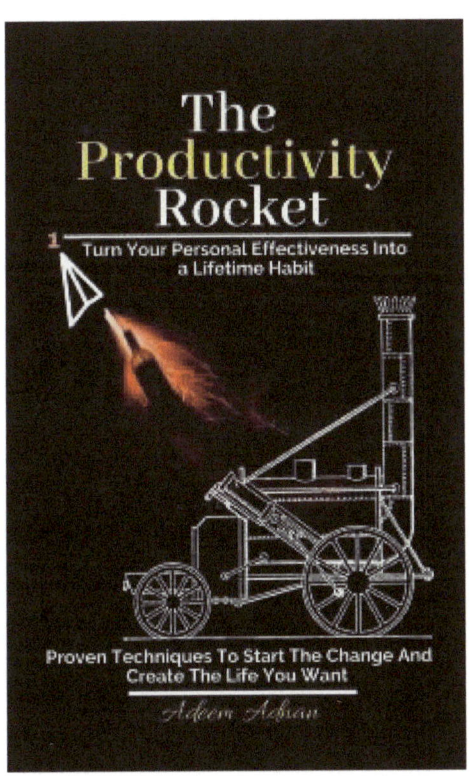

---

clarifying purposes only and are the owned by the owners themselves, not affiliated with this document.

★★★★★

This book dedicated to everybody has decided to taste the change in their life.

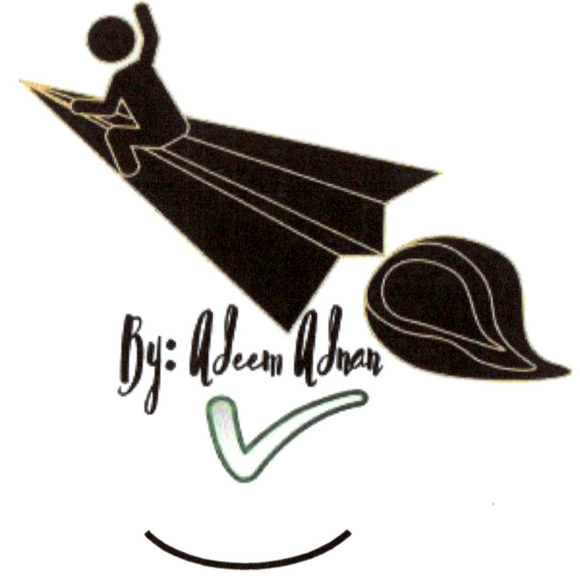

Table of Contents:

Introduction: --------------------

ChapterI: See The Big Picture.

ChapterII: Make Every Action Count

ChapterIII:How They Work!

ChapterIV: Some Keys you need to understand

Conclusion: ---------------------

<u>**Introduction:**</u>

Why should you read this book? This book is a collection of important productivity boosting techniques I've tried and tested throughout the years. The transitioning from working full time for others to being a full time online business owner is not easy at all.

I was challenged on so many levels. The information you will read in this book focuses on the productivity habits that I actually developed... and kept. This is not theory. This book does not contain stuff that I haven't tried. If I list a method here, it is because I have not only tried it, but it has worked for me.

It's fairly easy to change your routine to adopt a new habit. The problem lies in getting that habit to stick. If you've ever tried to lose weight, you know exactly what I'm talking about. One key discovery I learned in my personal journey of trying one habit after another is the importance of building systems.

If you were to build new habits just by picking up an "efficiency hack" here and there, you won't hang on to those habits. How come? Your other habits or routines don't reinforce them. It's as if you just picked up a hack or a more efficient way of doing things, but as soon as your situation changes, you forget all about them. You did not incorporate them into your lifestyle. Often, you'd even forget what to do to boost your overall productivity and efficiency.

This book helps you to build a system of habits which reinforce each other. The more habits you add on, the harder it would be for you to forget your existing habits. It's as if you've completely changed key parts of your life. Excited yet? Let's dive in.

Chapter 1: See the big picture Act out of purpose

A lot of people try to change their lives for the better. In fact, the global weight loss industry is a multi-billion dollar industry precisely for this reason. People are unhappy with who they see in the mirror. This is why there are all sorts of self-improvement and weight loss programs all over the world.

Sadly, most people who try to change their lives at one level or other meet with failure, If not immediately, eventually. What's wrong? A lot of them, I would say most of them, can't sustain their drive for change.

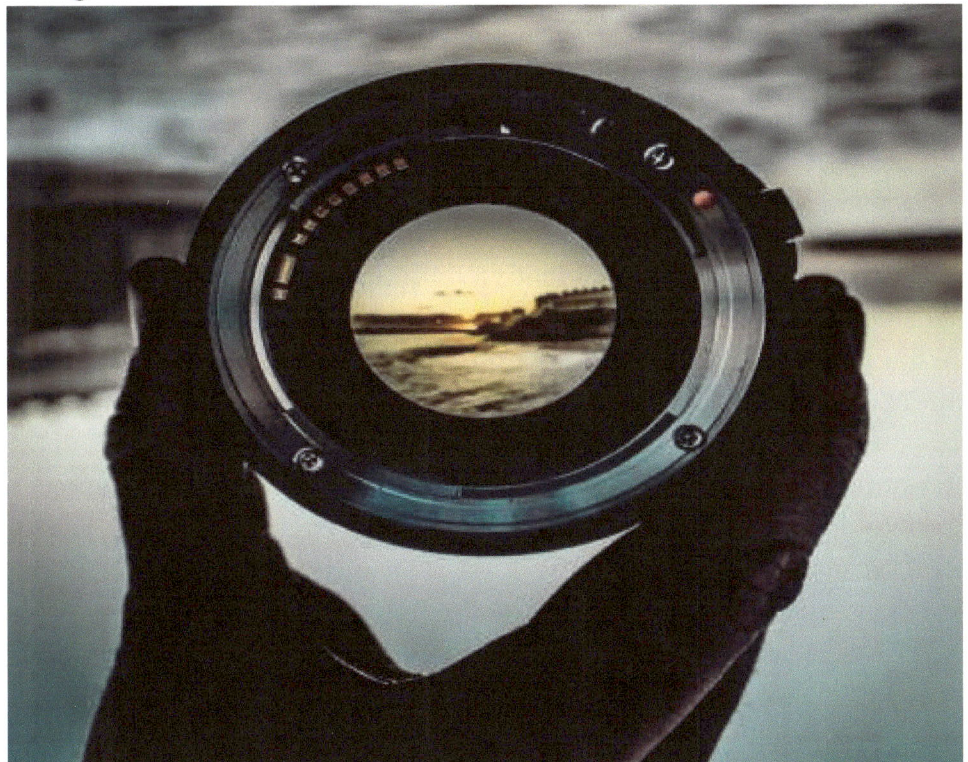

Let me tell you, nothing will wake you up faster than just looking in the mirror and seeing that you need to change. Maybe you got sick and tired of not getting promoted at work. Maybe you're unhappy with the low pay check you take home every two weeks.

Whatever it is you are frustrated with, chances are there came a point that you truly wanted to change. It's as if the moment of truth arrived. Welcome to the club. Almost everybody I know experiences that at one point in their life.

The problem is as pumped up and as excited as we are to change, eventually, our passion dies away. It's as if the rest of our lives catch up to us and we end up where we began. I know this sounds sad, right? Here's one solution that worked for me: Focus on your life's grand objective.

When I looked at being more productive as a simple tool that I can use so I can make more money, I got pumped up. I have to admit, I was excited for a few weeks, but eventually, my old routines kicked in. My old habits got the better of me and I went back to where I started.

I was only able to get lasting results when I stopped looking at increasing my personal productivity and being a better time manager as ends in of themselves. Instead, I looked at my life's grand objective. What kind of life am I trying to build for myself? What did I want from life?

I wanted a life that I could be proud of. I wanted a life marked by concrete achievements that I can proudly say were mine. When I shifted my focus from what was five feet in front of me to the grand purpose of my life, things began to change. From that point on, my habits were not just about "being more efficient." My mindset was not trained on just saving time.

When I looked at these grand objectives, I discovered my life's purpose. It really shocked me when I discovered that my life purpose is not just about becoming rich. It really opened my eyes when I realized that my life purpose is not just about getting promoted at work or getting that prestigious corner office.

It dawned on me that my life purpose highlights my character, values and what truly is important to me. This is not a philosophical experiment. This truly changed how I thought about myself and how I went about doing things. I realized that when I focus on my life's purpose, my goals had to align with them. If they didn't, I was wasting my time.

This really opened my eyes to many areas of my life that I was neglecting. I started acting with purpose. This meant I was more motivated. Most importantly, this meant I remained motivated at all times.

How come? Well, everything I do makes sense to me. Everything I do leads to my purpose or it doesn't. That's why I make a clear choice.

Be Clear About Your Grand Objectives

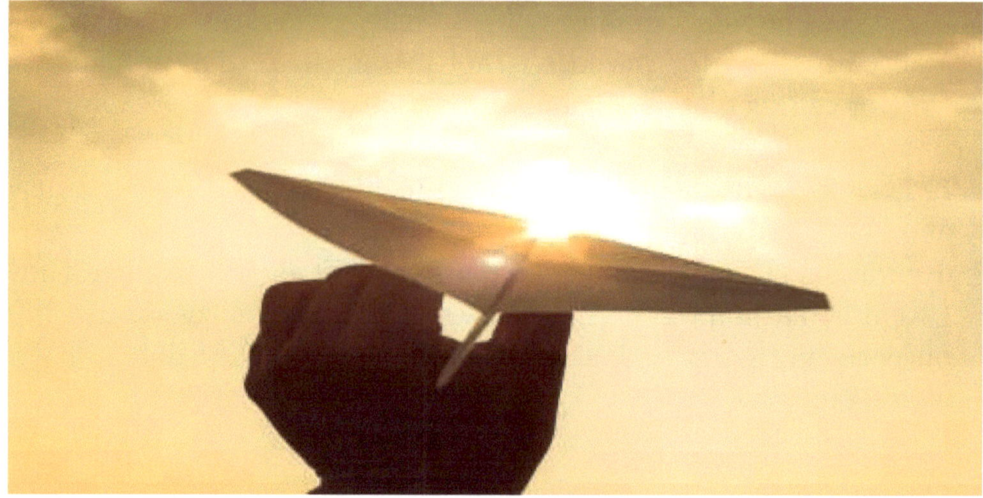

If you want to be more effective and productive person, focus on the grand objective of your life. Look past the dollar signs. Look past the big house, the nice cars and the prestige.

What exactly do you want to achieve with your life?

This is a very big question that most people assume they have the answer to. That is the reason why they continue to struggle. They assume that they already have a grand objective. Accordingly, it does not line up with how they behave. It doesn't give them the energy they need to become more productive on a day to day basis.

You have to be clear about the fact that how you do things now doesn't lead to your grand objective. The reason why you're struggling and are frustrated in many areas of your life is because of a disconnect. That's right. There is a disconnect between the grand purpose and objective of your life and how you choose to do things.

Does any of this sound familiar? Do you spend a lot of energy on all sorts of tasks every single day? But if you are able to knock them out and accomplish them, you realize you're no closer to your grand objectives. Does this happen to you? Do you put a lot of time into all sorts of things but you end up no closer to your dreams? Do you happen to achieve certain goals but somehow, these goals don't get you any closer to your grand objectives in life?

If any of that applies to you, then there is a disconnect in your life. You're not living purposefully. You're not living intentionally. You don't have a guiding light or a map in front of you. Instead, you just spend a tremendous amount of time, effort and energy in the dark. It's as if you were chasing your tail.

This has nothing to do with the amount of energy you put in to your activities. This has nothing to do with how well you know how to do things. The problem is the obstacle lies in HOW you pursue the why of your life.

You focus on how to do things. It never occurred to you that you have a very fuzzy or unclear picture of why you're doing what you're doing. Again, this is beyond getting enough money to pay the rent. This goes far beyond trying to get rich. Understand the why of your life.

If you can get an answer and you're not happy with it, there's good news for you. You can always choose a different purpose. You can clarify your life's purpose. You can redirect or revise it. It doesn't matter whether you just graduated from high school and are starting your life or you just graduated from college or graduate school. It doesn't matter if you're 80 years old. You can still clarify the grand objectives of your life and let go of objectives that you may have been pursuing but doesn't fit the values that you want for yourself.

Fix these grand objectives and you would be able to let go of obstacles that block how you will achieve your grand objective. Do you see the relationship between the "how" and "why"? These have to fit. The reason why you're struggling is because how you choose to do things doesn't line up with why you're doing things.

You're grand objective doesn't flow logically to what you're doing in the here and now. If you're able to line these up, you'll be able to act out of purpose. You become more motivated to clear obstacles in your way. Your number one goal is to reach your grand objective. This is why you will be able to see and knock out obstacles like bad time management, time wasting habits, inefficient problem solving and hanging on to counterproductive habits.

*****

<u>**Chapter 2:**</u> **Make every action count**

But it all starts with the moment of clarity. Be clear about the grand objective in your life. Ask yourself, "What do I want from my life?" All the answers flow from this question.

Now that you're clear about your life's grand objective, the next step is to tie these to goals. Please understand that your grand objective is different from your goals. Goals are actionable plans that enable you to turn your grand life objectives into reality.

Let's put it this way, grand life objectives without goals are simple day dreams. There's a big difference. When you're daydreaming, you're not planning to achieve what you're dreaming about. Instead, you're escaping. You're unhappy with your life. So what do you do?

Instead of lifting a finger to change your practical reality, you imagine yourself in a different time, place and life. When you daydream, you waste all the emotional urgency of wanting to change your present reality for the cheap "emotional high" of hopes and wishes that you know will never become reality. You waste energy and precious time when you do this. You have to set goals. Goals are what separate daydreams from grand life objectives.

Let me let you in on a secret about goals.

What if I told you that with effective goal setting, nothing is impossible? Don't believe me? Well, it's not your goal that makes it impossible. It's the timeline you give yourself. You only need to look at the US moon mission to understand this

When President Kennedy declared to the world that after a few years, there will be a man on the moon, a lot of people thought he was crazy. These critics had a lot going for them. Why? When Kennedy made that announcement, the technology didn't exist to put people on the moon.

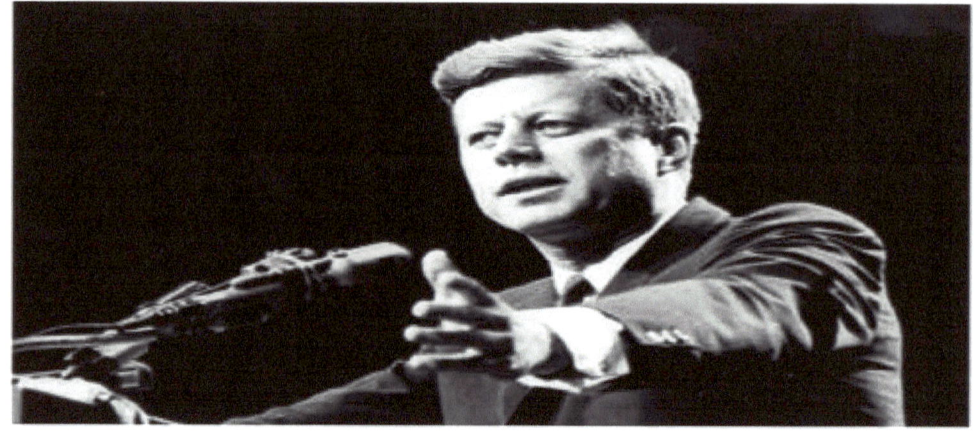

https://patch.com/massachusetts/boston/ask-not-what-twitter-can-do-you-jfk-logs

Still, by the time 1969 rolled around, the technology existed. It is not the goal that makes it impossible. It's the timeline. In NASA's case, the technology evolved by a certain date so they were able to deliver on President Kennedy's goal.

The grand objective was to put a man on the moon. This was broken down into big goals. These big goals were then broken down into smaller chunks. For example, if you're going to put a man on the moon, you're going to have to develop better rockets. This means you're going to have to develop better rocket fuel.
This also requires better navigation and the design of a re-entry vehicle. This also means you have to set a goal of developing space suits that would withstand the pressures of gravity-free space.

In other words, NASA took the big objective of President Kennedy and broke it down into big goals. It then broke down those big goals to smaller chunks.

As each goal gets smaller and smaller, they become easier to achieve. How come? They become less intimidating. Let me tell you, if you were in 1960 and somebody told you "I want your program to send a man on the moon" you would think that that person is crazy. You might even be tempted to say that it's impossible.

But when you start breaking down that grand objective into big goals and each big goal is broken down into practical sub-goals, it's no longer intimidating. You start thinking in terms of practical questions like "What kind of fuel is needed to beat the earth's gravity? What kind of material is needed to keep an astronaut safe while in outer space?"

You start thinking in terms of these practical questions. Gone is the intimidation of "OMG, you're telling me I must put a man on the moon!" When you break down your big goals into smaller chunks, you start focusing on specific actions. This, in turn, can be plugged into a routine.

What if I told you that NASA did not have easy answers in the beginning, but they had many different alternative answers this was their process. Selecting among different options was part of their routine. When you plug in these smaller sub goals into your routine, the answer appears sooner rather than later. This process doesn't just apply to NASA. It applies to you as well.

Break down sub-goals into daily or periodic to-do list items

Now that you know what your big goals are and broken them down into sub-goals, turn those sub-goals into daily or periodic to-do list items. The daily items are tasks that you do every day. Periodic items, on the other hand, are sub-goal tasks that you do at specific times or periods.

For example, after you have put in a week of your daily tasks, then you do one of your periodic tasks, maybe it involves some sort of quality control or it may involve selling whatever you produce for the week. Whatever the case may be, this sub-goal task is something that you don't do every day. It is usually dependent on the tasks that you do daily.

Making every action count

Your to-do list must directly tie to your sub-goals. Just by looking at your to-do list, you must clearly see how they make your sub-goals possible.

 Next, when you look at your sub-goals, you can easily piece them together and figure out the big goal you're trying to achieve.

Finally, when you look at your big goals, you must easily see that they lead to your grand objectives. If there is a disconnect here or you can't see the connection, then there's a problem. Maybe that to-do list item doesn't really take you to your grand objective.

You have to look at the whole picture. Everything must lead to your grand objectives; otherwise, that activity doesn't belong on your schedule.

By insisting on that tight connection, you will stop working on pointless tasks. Every little bit counts. Also, it becomes so much easier for you to get and stay motivated. Why? Everything leads to your life changing. Everything leads to the work of your life.

How long will it take to develop new habits?

This book will teach you how to develop habits so you can become more productive. These productivity habits will lead you to your grand objectives. Indeed, it is these objectives that give you the passion and focus you need to take care of your daily tasks.

Developing habits can take as little as 21 days or as much as 60 days or beyond. It really depends on you. It depends on how motivated you are and how stable your situation is. The more unstable your schedule or your circumstances, the more time you have to give yourself to adopt these habits.

Still, time is on your side. It doesn't really matter whether it will take you 21 days or 60 days. You need to stick to these tasks and process until they sink in.

Should you replace bad habits?

A lot of people have a tough time adopting good habits because they feel they have to replace bad habits. What if I told you that you don't have to do that? What if I told you that picking up new productivity habits is actually easier than you think!

How? Displace your old habits. In other words, focus on adding new habits instead of actively killing your old habits. Usually, when you adopt a new habit that offsets or cancels out an existing habit, the old habit will just go away. Focus on your new habits. Focus on adding them. Don't waste precious time and energy trying to actively replace your existing habits.

*****

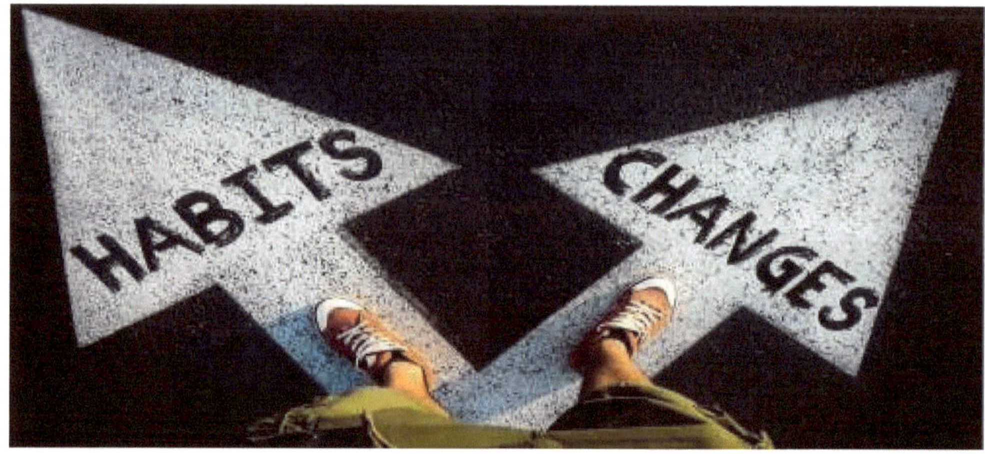

Habits have **3 components**. A lot of people think that habits all boil down to the action somebody automatically makes. For example, if you see somebody at the bar and they only need to walk in and order a drink and they would start drinking. A lot of people think that this is all there is to alcoholism. That's not true.

The same goes with smoking. A lot of people think that nicotine addicts basically just want to light up. You're only looking at the habitual action portion of habits. Habits can actually have 3 components. All 3 must be present otherwise, the habit will not stick.

It doesn't matter whether we're talking about good habits or bad ones. These 3 components must always be present.

Trigger

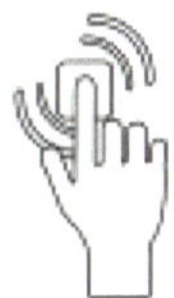

All habits require a trigger. This is the stimulus that tells your body that you should engage in habitual action if you want to get the reward that you are accustomed to. These triggers can be physical. For example, if you're a smoker, you usually get triggered after eating a meal or if you're waiting in line somewhere and you're bored. These physical triggers push you to light up or whip out a vape device. The truth is, people get triggered by other things. You can be triggered by thoughts, other people or time. For example, if you have a habit of lighting up first thing in the morning, your alarm clock might go off and that's when you know it's time to head outside for a quick smoke. Similarly, your smoking habit may be attuned to your body clock. So by the time 5am rolls around, you get out of bed and light up. You are triggered by time.

Habitual action

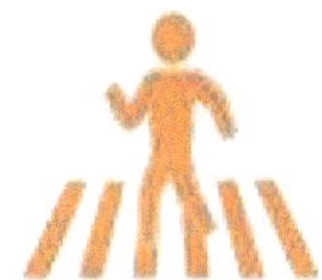

This is the part of habits that is easy to understand. This is the action that you take. Please understand that this does not necessarily mean physical action. It can also mean mental action.

For instance, if you have a bad relationship with your father and you remember a certain incident in your childhood, that mental image is enough to depress you, throw you into a fit of rage or otherwise impact your emotions negatively.

Your father may have died a long time ago, but you still get triggered into habitual mental action by this person's memory.

Habitual action can also involve speech. For instance, if a friend of yours tells you that she saw somebody you knew from high school, maybe this would trigger you to gossip about that person or people who know that person.

Reward

What if I told you that habits would not be formed if there was no reward? You may be shocked. A lot of people think that people develop habits because they get physically hooked on some substance. It's easy to look at alcoholism and nicotine addiction from this perspective.

But it's actually more than that. When you take habitual action, you do that because you are looking for some sort of reward at the end of the process. It doesn't have to be some sort of biochemical reaction like you would get with smoking, drinking or doing drugs.
It can be a physical rush. For instance, people who have developed a healthy addiction to running or jogging first thing in the morning get a nice physical rush thanks to endorphins. Similarly, if you get triggered and you start gossiping, you get that emotional state of feeling superior or feeling like you are letting other people in on a secret that only you know.
That emotional rush that you get, That's a reward. Other people engage in habits because they want a certain physical or emotional state of mind. Others do it for money. Whatever the case may be, there has to be some sort of reward. This is what cements the connection between the trigger and habitual action.

Turbocharge habit formation by focusing on your purpose

When you focus on the grand objectives of your life and you tie them into what you need to do when you detect certain triggers, your life goes to another level. You're more likely to do things that you normally would want to avoid on time, every time.

Instead of screwing around at work, checking your Facebook updates, social media accounts or email for the millionth time, you focus on what your boss is paying you to do. Just as importantly, when you focus on your purpose, your habits are likely to stick.
You're more motivated. You realize that there is a point to your habitual actions. They lead to somewhere big and important. You're not just chasing your tail or wasting time.

You eventually realize that working towards your life's purpose is your ultimate reward. That's right. This is better than the emotional rush of judging other people when you're gossiping. This is far superior to the chump change you make working a little harder. This is much better than whatever physical high you get smoking, drinking or doing drugs.

Working towards your purpose and seeing that purpose turn from idea to a reality you can see, touch, taste, smell and hear is the ultimate reward. Why? You know full well very few people get to that point.

Your Productivity Habit Road Map

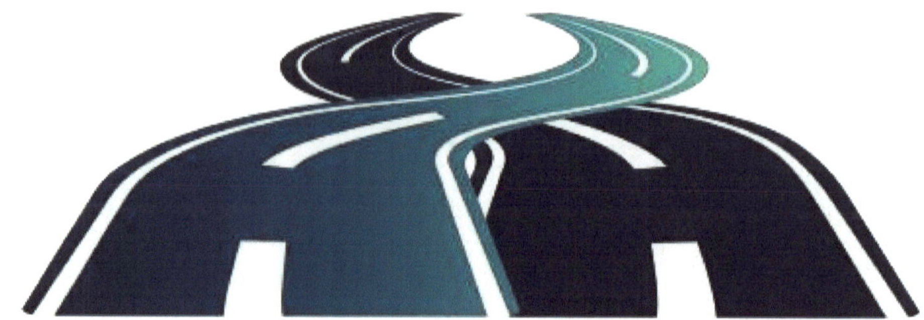

What follows is a step by step guide to the habits that you need to adopt to become extremely productive. Please understand that this is not going to happen overnight. Don't expect to explode your productivity on day 1. These habits take quite some time to sink in. However, once you have established one habit, it's so much easier to establish the second habit and then the third and fourth.

This is the difference between a habit system where each subsequent habit reinforces existing habits and hacks. Some productivity hacks are necessary, but don't get the 2 confused. You need to develop habits. These are what will see you through.

Hacks often depend on your mood. They often depend on circumstances beyond your control. Your habits, on the other hand, can see you through even if you don't feel like it. Even if you woke up on the wrong side of the bed, the right habits can ensure that you do what you need to do when you need to do it to maximize your personal productivity.

Follow the road map below. Please feel free to tweak and make small adjustments so they fit your particular set of circumstance.

Habit #1 Read your list of grand objectives and your goals

It's really important to have a clear idea of what your life's grand objectives are. Once you have this down in writing, write down the goals that lead to those grand objectives. Your trigger is time. Do this first thing in the morning and late at night, hopefully before you get to bed.

The reward you get when you adopt this habit is a sense of mental and emotional clarity. You quickly realize that despite whatever drama is happening in your life that there is this giant light in the middle. You just need to follow that light because that is what your life is about.

These are your grand objectives. There are specific stones that you have to step on to get to that light. These are your goals. This is a tremendous sense of mental relief. How come? Just simply compare it to what you were doing before.

Before, you were probably just trying to keep your head above water. You were struggling and flailing. And often end up chasing your tail.

Habit #2 Plan your day the night before

List out your to-do list and prioritize them. I'm not talking about prioritizing them in terms of how easy they are to knock out. This is not about convenience. Instead, list them out in terms of importance measured by how important they are in helping you achieve your goals which lead to your grand objectives.

Again, everything you do must have a direct line or link to the grand objectives of your life. This includes your daily to-do list. You have to do this the night before. Your trigger is time. The ideal time for this an hour or so before bed time.

I want you to develop this habit so that when you sense that you're going to sleep in about an hour or so, you whip out a notepad and start listing out your to-do list for the next day. Once you have put together your list, you then prioritize or sort the list depending on importance as far as your life's objectives are concerned.

The reward that you get is a strong sense of purpose. You get a sense that you are doing something concrete to move your life in the right direction. When you realize this, you can't help but feel motivated and pumped up. You say to yourself, "I am going places. I'm doing the right things. I have purpose."

Habit #3 Practice gratitude for a few minutes every morning

You don't have to be a spiritual, mystical or religious person, but a little bit of gratitude goes a long way. When you practice gratitude, you either list down or simply think about the things that are going right in your life.

It doesn't have to be big, but list down everything that you're aware of. For example, if you've ever suffered from kidney stones, that incident will let you know the importance of healthy kidneys. How often do you take your kidneys for granted?

Write down everything that you can be thankful for. Write down that you are thankful to be alive, that you're breathing normally, that you don't have cancer. Don't focus on the things that you don't have. Focus on the things that you do have.

Spoiler alert: If you live in the US or any other "developed country," you are in the top 10% of the globe's population. What if I told you hundreds of millions of people on the planet get by on less than a dollar a day. Let that sink in.

Find something to be grateful for. Your trigger is time. You need to do this first thing in the morning. Maybe right after the alarm clock rings or right after you pop out of bed. Whatever the case may be, prepare your mind for a day of explosive productivity by choosing to be grateful.

The reward that you get is a sense of possibility. You get excited about your day. You also get rid of stress. The awesome thing about practicing gratitude is that it shifts your mental focus from how scary, intimidating and problematic certain tasks are and you focus on what you have. You focus on possibility. You focus on what's going well.

This goes a long way in eliminating stress and giving you much needed perspective.

Habit #4 Exercise in the morning

I don't care what you physically do in the morning as long as it gets your blood pumping and gets fresh air in your lungs, you should do it. Maybe you can only walk around the block. That's fine. Maybe you can jog to a nearby park. That would be awesome. Maybe you can bike several miles a day. That will be plenty.

Whatever the case may be, get physical exercise. It can even be tai chi as long as you know how to do it right. The trigger here, of course, is time. You have to set a specific time in the morning. Maybe you could set up an alarm clock. Do this right after you practice gratitude.

The reward that you get is a combination of both physical and mental benefits. When you work out, you become physically pumped up. You get a lot more energy because you have a lot more oxygen circulating through your system.

This leads to mental benefits because oxygen reinvigorates your brain. You become mentally awake. This leads to both mental and physical energy.

Habit #5 don't weigh yourself down with a heavy breakfast

This is where a lot of people stumble. They wake up all pumped up, they follow habits 1-4 to the letter, but they treat themselves to heavy meals. I'm talking about heavy carbohydrate meals. Maybe they load up on the pancakes, bread, pasta, mashed potatoes or rice.
Whatever form it takes, when you load up with a heavy breakfast, you are actually setting yourself up for a big letdown for the rest of the day. Instead of feeling like you're on top of the world and you can take care of whatever challenges life throws your way, you feel weighed down.

This is why you should focus on eating mostly protein and some fat. Try to cut out as much carbs as possible. Keep high carbohydrate food at a minimum. I'm not saying you should cut them out completely, but try to cut back because you want to feel light yet energized. High protein and a little bit of fat will do the trick.

The trigger for this habit is time. Obviously, you have to do this during breakfast time. The reward you get is unmistakable. You feel pumped up. You feel light and flexible. This gives you the ability to adapt to whatever the day has in store for you.

Habit #6 Knock out your to-do list part 1

Whether you go to a home office or you go to a nearby corner cafe or you go to a formal office to do your work, you need to knock out your to-do list in 2 parts. This is part 1.

When you decide to work, focus on your to-do list and drill down that list. In other words, since you sorted your list in terms of priority, go down the list in order. Don't look for the "easy stuff." Follow the order.

If the first item is the toughest, then so be it. Knock it out. Devote all your early morning will power and focus on the hardest things first because these are the ones that lead to your grand life objective.

The trigger here is the time. You do this in the morning. Also, this trigger must be matched with a place. Get triggered by the fact that you sat down in front of your computer. This is show time. Once you detect that it's morning and you have sat down in front of your computer and it's time to work. Drill down on your list with full power and focus knocking out item after item.

What is the reward that you get? You get a nice surge of emotional clarity and a distinct thrill when you overcome the initial "blockage" that you normally experience. Let's face it, usually, you feel a sense of hesitation or there's some sort of mental block when you look at your to-do list.

Normally, you would look for the easiest parts first and then worry about the harder stuff. Unfortunately, it's the hard stuff that actually pushes your life forward. When you resolve to knock out your to-do list in order, you get that great release. You realize, "I can do these stuff. I've done it before and now, I have not let my fear intimidate me."

The more you do this and experience that sense of great release, the less likely you would feel blocked early in the morning. Little by little, all the initial intimidation goes away. Eventually, this can turn into such a habit that the moment you get into your office and look at your to-do list, you jump right in and knock out the hardest item in that list and blast through task list item after item like a hot knife cutting through butter.

You do this with an expectation of that awesome reward of that sense of great release and relief that you feel as you knock out each item.

Habit #7: Cut out the noise

When you're doing your work, focus on doing work. This means that you have to develop the habit of absolutely cutting out whatever noise you normally encounter. I'm talking about checking for social media updates and emails or talking to people at work and around you. I'm also talking about you checking your phone. You have to cut all that out. That is noise!

When you sit down to do work, get to work. Focus on the great sense of release that you get when you knock out to do list item after item. The trigger for cutting out noise is time and place. The time usually is the morning, and you're triggered by a sense of place when you sit down in front of your computer. You remain focused on knocking out one task after another. This means that the reward you're looking for is an uninterrupted sense of release, power, and relief.

Habit #8: Stick to fixed break schedules

If you work for somebody else, by law, they have to give you an hour lunch break and two 15-minute breaks. Stick to that schedule. Keep one hour lunches exactly one hour and 15-minute breaks exactly 15 minutes. The trigger here is your clock. Once it's lunch time, go to lunch. Once the time is over, get back to work.

Your reward here is the sense that no energy is lost when you break for meals. Your focus is where it needs to be. When you are working, your focus is on work. When you're on lunch break, your focus can be on something else. By sticking to this fixed schedule, you feel recharged and most importantly you feel in control. You don't feel sidetracked, you don't feel disoriented, and you don't feel like you have all these pressures going on. Instead, you feel in control because you know when to stop and start working.

Habit #9: Use your breaks to get a big picture view of your tasks

During your break, look at what you're doing. In particular, eat, sit back, relax and calmly think about all your tasks in context. Why are you doing what you're doing? Where do they all lead to? If you follow this blueprint properly, they all lead to your grand objective.

If you can see that tight connection, you can't help but feel pumped up and excited. The trigger, this happens after your meal, after having some coffee or sipping some tea. Allow yourself to enter a contemplative state of mind. The reward that you get is a sense of calm and focus. You also can get a sense of accomplishment or an anticipation of what's happening next. You also are more likely to get a sense of excitement over solving problems that lay in the way of your grand objective.

Compare this with the normal, emotional, and mental states of people during their lunch break. They think about a sense of having skipped the ordeal of their work. They hate their jobs so much and they think it's so pointless. Now they're getting a nice little break. It's their oasis, it's little moment of calm. But this sense of calm is a sense of avoidance and relief from work.

The reward that you're looking for is the precise opposite. It involves calm, but it also involves a sense of accomplishment because you ran towards your work instead of running away from it.

The sense of accomplishment you get is when you knock out work and achieve goal after goal on your way to the grand objectives of your life.

Big difference, Is not it?

Habit #10: Knock out your to do list Part 2

By this point you've gone back to work. You then resume what you were doing before. This means drilling down on your to do list in order. The trigger here is time. This happens after each break. The reward is again, the sense that you've overcome an initial blockage or resistance. You get that sense great release of energy and focus. You also look forward to the increasing levels of energy and motivation as you destroy one task list item after another.

Habit #11: Learn to say no

Understand that throughout the typical workday, there will be a lot of people asking stuff from you that is not directly related to your to do list. This is a problem, especially if this person is your boss.
 It's really important to know how to say no. You have to sort the things they're telling you to do for them. Is it important and is it urgent? These are the two main considerations you should keep in mind.

If they're asking you to do something that is highly important and is urgent, do it, right then and there. If they're asking you to do something that is not all that important, but is urgent, do it, but look to delegate or even outsource that work. Depending on your job, you may be able to do this. If they're asking you to do something that is highly important, but is not urgent, you can either schedule this or defer it. Maybe you can put it in a future to do list. Finally, if you are being asked to do something that is not important and not urgent, you can either delegate this to somebody else, outsource it, postpone it, or forget it altogether.

The trigger in learning to say no is situational. It's time based. It doesn't happen all the time and it depends on the situation. The reward that you get when you learn this habit is that you stay focused on your price. You cherish that fact and get a sense of victory because you were able to overcome a fairly hard challenge. Sometimes it's very hard to say no.

Habit #12: Recognize when you enter "states of flow"

A state of flow is when everything comes easy to you. For example, if you are a professional writer and you normally stumble the first few minutes trying to write an article. When you enter a state of flow, you are able to blast through one article after another. You are able to handle the twists and turns of your daily work with ease. Even if you start handling more difficult tasks, they don't feel heavy.

You are able to move quickly, produce more, and most importantly stick to your quality standards. Ultimately, this habitual action climaxes with a massive rush of a sense of a mastery. You feel that you're good at something. You feel that you're an expert on something. This is priceless.

The trigger for this habitual action is a prolonged series of finishing to do list items at high quality levels. When you go through your to do list and you knock out one item after another, eventually you realize that the you are able to maintain your quality. This makes it more and more apparent to you that you have achieved a state of flow. The reward that you get is a feeling of momentum. It's as if the world cannot stop you. You also gain a tremendous surge of confidence from an increasing awareness of your personal competence.

Let me be clear. Forget about what you've heard. In the United States, the whole "self-esteem" movement is very big. According to this movement you have to build up kids' self-esteem so that they would become more self-confident, which can lead to them doing better work. This is not true. That movement actually has the process in reverse.

When you get good at something, you become more self-confident and then, you're able to experiment and do more things to take your game to a much higher level. You become even more competent, which leads to an even higher level of confidence. Don't confuse the two. Nowhere in this process do you start with self-esteem. Instead, you start with competence. By recognizing your states of flow, you gain a sense of competence which leads to increasing levels of confidence.

*****

<u>Chapter 4:</u> key Productivity Hacks: you need to understand

Use the following hacks to process your tasks faster without suffering any loss in output quality.

Hack #1: Find the familiar and get confident

If you're doing a new task, find parts of it that you have done before.

Here's the good news, even if your boss gives you a brand new project, chances are when you look at the actual processes involved in completing the project, 50% or more involve tasks that you've done before. Look for these. These are familiar to you. Allow yourself to feel assured that you're not doing something completely different or new. Let the feeling sink in.

Focus on the emotional state where you can say to yourself, "I've done this before and I can do it again", "It's fun scaling up what I've learned before", and "This is improving my expertise". When you're able to say these things to yourself, you get that sense of confidence that arises from competence. As you become familiar with the new project and are able to produce more and more results, your competence increases and boosts your confidence, which in turn enhances your competence. It's an upward spiral of personal mastery.

Hack #2: Think in terms of templates

If you're doing a task that has some familiar parts, do what you did in the past and fill in the template. In other words, do the things that are familiar to you and then fill in the unknown parts. When you do this, you're not reinventing the wheel. You're also freeing yourself from the unnecessary intimidation and fear of having to "learn something new". By focusing on the familiar and using your past work on them as some sort of "template", you will be able to get out from under whatever emotional intimidation new or big tasks normally bring.

Hack #3: Run a race with yourself

Break down your tasks into small bite-sized chunks and time yourself completing each part.

Race with yourself. Note how long it takes doing one part and try to beat your previous time while maintaining the same quality. Keep doing this until you're able to knock out all the small chunks related to that specific task. The best part of all of this is you get rid of whatever emotional intimidation and fear you may have had about your project.

Hack #4: Try to break stuff as you work on your tasks

Explore different software options for your tasks, if your work provides it. Do the different tasks involved in the specific to do list item in a different order. When you do this, you're conducting experiments so you can see if there is some sort of shortcut. Use whatever you can find and see if you can do more in less time. This will enable you to produce a lot more or free up enough time so you could increase your output quality.

Hack #5: Record your shortcuts and productivity lessons

Whenever you do anything, you learn how to do things the regular way and the enhanced way. If you're doing a task that you've done before, there's a good chance that you may come up with an enhancement or an improvement.

Unfortunately, you cannot just enjoy that brainstorm and then forget it by tomorrow. If you really want to take your productivity to the next level, document or write down your brainstorms. It doesn't have to be the very best idea in the world. Just document everything.

If you follow the hack above, you're going to be running all sorts of experiments. Read through your documentation and remind yourself of the lessons you learned. When you do this, you'll be able to connect the dots and apply these experiments that boost your productivity or work quality. Eventually, you will be able to do both.

Good Luck

*****

Success is a habit. It really is. It's not something that just dropped in the laps of successful people. They didn't just stumble upon it. In all likelihood, they themselves changed on their journey to success. You have to change as well. You have to build a habit system where each habit reinforces each other. This is the key to becoming an unstoppable learning machine on your way to achieving the grand objectives of your life.

Let all your actions be guided by purpose and you will be able to adopt all twelve productivity habits that will take your life to the next level.

I wish you nothing but an incredible success

If you've enjoyed this book or found it useful I'd be very grateful if you'd post a short review on Amazon. Your support really does make a difference and I read all the reviews personally so I can get your feedback and make this book even better and better. If you'd like to leave a review then all you need to do is click the review link on this book's page on Amazon here:

https://www.amazon.com/Productivity-Rocket-Personal-Effectivenes-techniques-ebook/dp/B07MDM5Y68

Scroll down the page, follow me and post your review
Your support is highly appreciated,

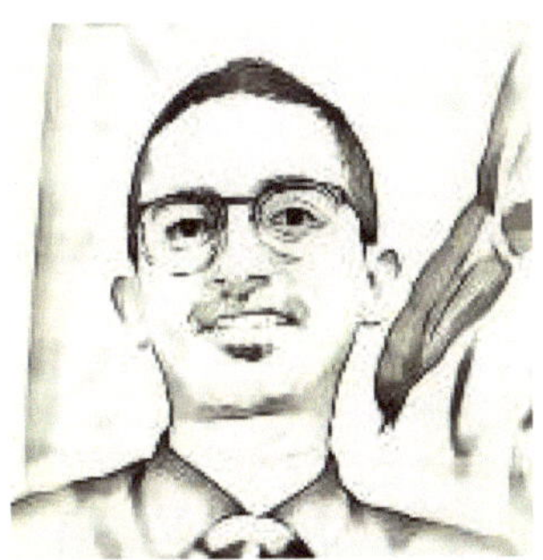

Adeem Adnan